Recipe for Happiness

# Recipe for happiness

## Jasmin Hajro

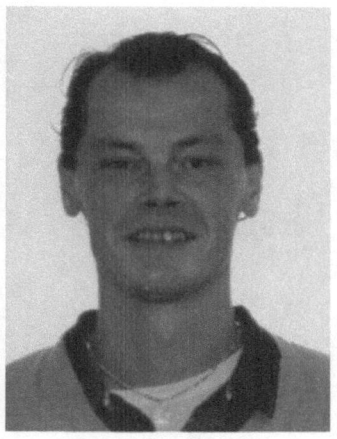

Jasmin Hajro

© 2018 Jasmin Hajro

ISBN : 978-0-244-39302-1

Cover design by

Jasmin Hajro

Second edition 2018

In this short booklet you will discover:

The bio of author Jasmin Hajro

&

book The Recipe for Happiness

&

A preview of book Build Your Fortune

&

A small acquaintance with establishment Hajro

## The bio of author Jasmin Hajro, nice to meet you

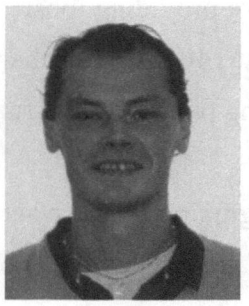

Hello dear reader,
how are you ?

Thank you for buying booklet Recipe for Happiness.

My name is Jasmin Hajro, I was born on July 6, 1985 in Bosnia.

As refugees, we came to the Netherlands 21 years ago.

After having completed school & worked at several jobs ...

On 17 December 2012, I founded my first company: investment firm Jasko.

After a successful first year, I unfortunately had to close that company.

After a short period of rest, unemployment and temporary work.

I started again as an entrepreneur.

On September 1, 2015, I founded establishment Hajro.

( We say establishment instead of company,
because we do a bit more then just sell stuff.
Like providing jobs,
donating to 40 different charities,
and helping people to live richer. )

Since the beginning the core activity is,
selling sets of greeting cards, door to door.
Nowadays the product range has been expanded.

With, among other things, the selling of my 10 books.

The royalties of my books are donated
to the charity: foundation Giveth Life.

My company is now part of Hajro Group,

which consists of 20 different subsidiaries,

that are part of 1 umbrella organization.

For more information about my company &
the foundation, go to www.hajrobv.nl

## The Recipe for Happiness

A book has been written about a true story ...
About a man who was imprisoned in a concentration camp
at the time of Hitler,
and happy.

So,
Happiness has nothing to do with your circumstances.

It has everything to do with,
your choice to be happy,
regardless of circumstances.

Choose to be happy.

Of course there are touhger times in life,
like when someone you love,
dies.
That's part of life.
Those times of grief you just have to go through and process.

Processing is best done by talking about it,
to get it off your chest regularly.

Or by writing about it,

if you write down a situation or your feelings about it,
then it's on paper,
and it is less in your head.
Writing is a good outlet.

Processing is also done well by:
staying busy.
Whether that is in your work or your hobby.
They say: a rolling stone does not collect moss.

So stay busy ....

Okay, now you have learned a good lesson about how to better process negative life experiences.

But you're here for the Recipe for Happiness, right?

Well, the lesson you've learned will help to make the recipe work better for you.

Here it comes then ...

You have probably read a local newspaper,

and you regularly check the news.

(the daily news on television)

Have you noticed that about 99% of it is bad news?
Only misery ..
If you did not know better,
you would think that the whole world is going to perish.

If it's a habit for you,
to watch the news every day for half an hour ...

Have you ever wondered if it's healthy for you?
Does it make you happy ?

Of course not !

The easiest way to change a habit is
by replacing it with a new habit.

So from today on,
instead of watching the worldly news
half an hour a day ..........

Watch COMEDY for half an hour a day.

Mandatory.

Every day.

Well, now at half past eight in the evening it's not news time,
but Comedy time.


If you watch comedy,
you relax &
you laugh.

Sounds healthier, doesn't it?

Well, laughing every day is easy to do, right?

And replacing your old bad habit in this way,
with a nice, healthy new habit,
is probably easier than you thought.

Except that relaxation is good for you,
when you laugh,
your body makes endorphins.

Those are natural happiness substances.

Well, after 21 days of daily watching comedy,
you will have formed a new habit.

So watch Comedy every day.

You can watch a lot of standup comedy on Youtube for free.

Simple?
Sure, but you have to do it,
every day,
until you don't have to think about it anymore,
and you start doing it automatically.

Some Happiness Ingredients in a row:

- Watch comedy every day, at least one hour.

- Eat ice cream, treat someone with an ice cream.

- Work out, throw out your frustration by playing tennis
or go for a run.

- Pee in the yard

(and if you get a fine for urinating, laugh your ass off)

- Do not worry, life is too short for that

(by staying busy, you do not have time to worry)

- Hug the people that you love

- Go enjoy a cup of coffee or tea

- Buy or save a cat or some other pet

- When you receive money, immediately save a part of it

- Don't let the media scare you,

the world is not getting worse, the world is getting better.

- Sex, need I say more

(when you have sex your body also produces endorphins = those natural happiness substances)

Maybe the Recipe for Happiness

is different than you had expected....

But that doesn't matter,

the point is that it works &

that it will help you to live happier.

Do it,

it is easier

then looking with a sour face.

If you liked this book & got some value from it.

Would you then be so kind,

please,

to recommend it

to the people that you know.

So that they too can enjoy it

and live happier.

Thank you very much.

———————————

It was my pleasure to write and translate

this book ( my third one )  for you.

I hope it helps you to live happier.

( I know it will, if you do the things it teaches )

And I hope, that we can together make a contribution

to more happiness in the world.

We can.
If you recommend this book
and share it.
Then I will promote it.

And together we will make a contribution to

a happier world.

I would appreciate it if you would write a short review.
Thank you for your effort.

Kind regards,

Jasmin Hajro

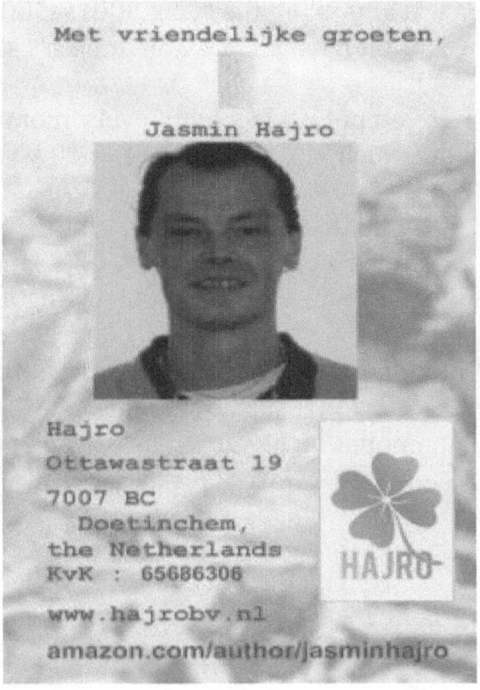

# Preview book Build your fortune

## the Pay yourself first principle

It means that when you receive your money,
you first pay yourself, by for example, setting aside a tenth.

To clarify your result,
we will make an example calculation.

For example, you earn 3000 euros or dollars per month.
And you pay yourself first,
in other words: you put aside a tenth (10%) of your income.
So you save 300, - euros per month.

A year has 12 months,
So after 1 year you'll have (12 x 300) = 3600, - euros.
After 1 year you have put a whole month's salary aside.

If you put aside a tenth every month,
how much will you have after 10 years?

(3600 x 10) = 36000, - euro.
So after 10 years you have 36000 euros
or a whole year's salary in your saving account.

Later on in this book: Build your Fortune,
you'll see how to make
that amount that you put aside each month.
Grow faster.

Preview book Build your Fortune

## 10% of everything

It is important that when you first pay yourself,
by setting aside 10%.
That you put 10% of everything aside.

Of course 10% of your income.

But also 10% of the tips if you receive any,

also 10% of your surtax,

also 10% of the money you receive as a gift,

also 10% of your 13th month,

also 10% of your bonus,

also 10% of your wage increase,

also 10% of your tax refund,

also 10% of your welcome bonus,

also 10% of your holidaypay.

No matter from which angle or from whom you receive money,
the first thing you do with it,
is to pay yourself first.
By setting aside a tenth of it.

End of preview.

Preview book Moneymaker

Moneymaker 3

The bible for entrepreneurs, written by an entrepreneur.
So your daily reading.

No, it's not about GOD.

It says, written by an entrepreneur .....

YOU READ ONLY BOOKS WHICH ARE WRITTEN BY PEOPLE WHO HAVE THEIR OWN COMPANY !!
Do you understand ?

This way you prevent feeding your mind with BULLSHIT.
And that you will model BULLSHIT.
So you save yourself time and money.

Ok, then a bit about that Entrepreneurial Bible.
It is called No Excuses, the Power of self discipline
And is written by Brian Tracy

And yes, he has his own company.
Otherwise his name would not be here.

It comes down to self discipline.
And self discipline makes you feel very good about yourself.


When you exercise, for example, while most people watch TV.
When you work on a Saturday, while most people have a weekend.
When you take a step towards achieving your goals on Sunday.

The above 3 examples require discipline from you.

But 1, 3, 5 years from now

where will you wind up ?

And where will most people wind up ?

Have you ever worked a day with pain because your teeth were broken?
Have you ever worked with only 2 hours of sleep, the night before?
Have you ever worked without having slept the night before?

It was probably easier to watch TV then .....

But if I did, then I would be a Bullshitter for you,
and not someone who you respect.

I disciplined my self and went to work.

Oh yeah, buy the entrepreneurial bible. NOW.

Previeuw book Moneymaker

Moneymaker 2.

Two things that you have to spend your time on daily

Which 2 are they?

Watch TV and be on Facebook?

Without B.S., so:

SALES & DIRECT MARKETING

If you sell something (sales), then profit comes in.

If you become good at (direct marketing), then profit comes in.

With marketing you save yourself time while selling.
You do not have to explain who you are and what your company does during your presentation.

How many hours per working day do you spend on sales?

How many hours per working day do You spend on Direct Marketing?

WHAT HAPPENS IF YOU ONLY SPEND YOUR WORKINGTIME ON SALES & DIRECT MARKETING ??

Will you have more profits and therefore more money?

End of preview
For more information about this book by me, go to
www.hajrobv.nl

## Small introduction with establishment Hajro

Establishment Hajro is committed to helping
the people in the province of Gelderland,
by providing jobs and keeping people working,
by donating to Charities,
and by helping people to live richer.

Today Hajro is
a subsidiary of Hajro Group.

The Hajro Group consists of 20 different companies,
who are all part of
1 umbrella organization.

We now have several products & services,
and we support more than 40 charities.

Visit us at www.hajrobv.nl

and discover what else we can do for you.

Hopefully you will become a raving fan & customer of us.

However you choose,

I wish you

a lot of prosperity & happiness.

Kind regards,

Jasmin Hajro

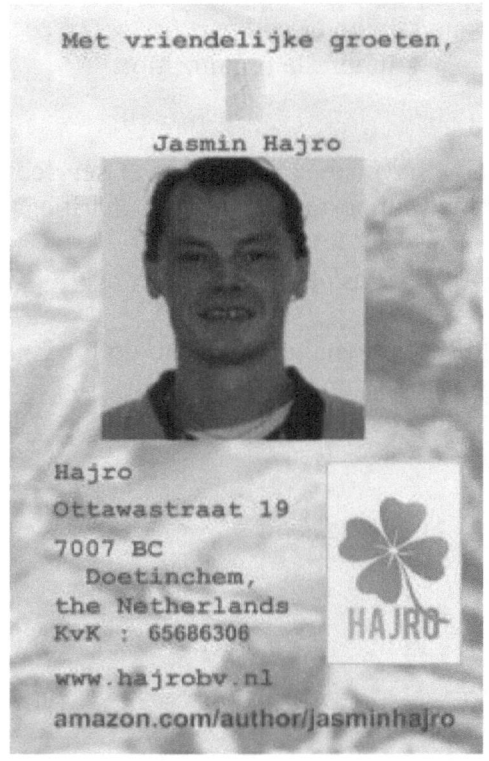

www.ingramcontent.com/pod-product-compliance
Lightning Source LLC
Chambersburg PA
CBHW020754230426
43665CB00009B/593